Liver Health

A Natural Approach

Martin Stone, M.H.

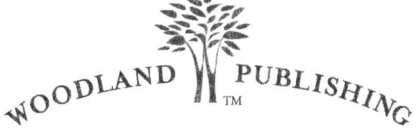

For permissions, ordering information, or bulk quantity discounts, please contact: Woodland Publishing, 448 East 800 North, Orem, Utah 84097
Visit our Web site: www.woodlandpublishing.com
Toll-free number: (800) 777-2665

The information in this book is for educational purposes only and is not recommended as a means of diagnosing or treating an illness. All matters concerning physical and mental health should be supervised by a health practitioner knowledgeable in treating that particular condition. Neither the publisher nor the author directly or indirectly dispenses medical advice, nor do they prescribe any remedies or assume any responsibility for those who choose to treat themselves.

Cataloging-in-Publication data available from the Library of Congress.

ISBN-13: 978-1-58054-397-2
ISBN-10: 1-58054-397-9

Printed in the United States of America

06   07   08   09   10   1   2   3   4   5   6   7   8   9   10

Contents

Introduction

The liver is one of the most important organs in the body because every substance that enters the body—either through the skin, the digestive system, or elsewhere—affects or is affected by the liver. So it's critical to ensure the proper functioning of this all-important but often-ignored organ.

This booklet will examine what the average person needs to do to maintain and cleanse the liver and the reasons why liver cleansing is one of the most important parts in maintaining good health.

The Liver

Your liver is located on the right side of your body directly under the diaphragm. It's about the size of your hand, and if you place your hand in front of your ribs on the right side of your body this is where your liver is located.

The liver is unusual in that it is both an organ and a gland. It is the largest gland and solid organ in the body and it differs in size from male to female. Women's livers weigh approximately 1.3 kilos, while men's weigh about 1.8 kilos.

At any given time, the liver contains a little over half a liter of blood and is estimated to have over five hundred different functions. Though your liver is unique in its ability to regenerate quickly and effectively, it can still be severely damaged by exposure to environmental toxins, drugs, and alcohol abuse. With over seventy thousand different chemicals in the food chain, it's imperative to regularly cleanse the liver to maintain optimal liver health.

The Four Basic Functions of the Liver

1. Liver cells continuously produce bilic acid and bile, which is one of our main digestive juices. Bile secretion from the liver also excretes toxins resulting from liver detoxification processes. Bile is stored and concentrated in the gallbladder, which is located just below the liver and then released into the small intestine as needed. Together, these organs process the nutrients found in the foods we eat. Without bile, about 40 percent of the fat we receive from foods would be lost in the stool, and the fat-soluble vitamins A, D, E, and K could not be absorbed. With bile, the fat we receive from food can be digested and absorbed in the small intestine.

2. The liver helps distribute and store the nutrients found in food. All animals use glucose that is stored in the liver to maintain blood-sugar levels within a very narrow parameter. This is of paramount importance in order to maintain energy levels and body functions, including brain function. This method of blood-sugar regulation evolved because, unlike humans, animals often don't eat on a regular basis. Regulation of blood glucose over varying amounts of time ranging from hours to weeks is needed to ensure energy levels that are crucial for survival.

The liver is the major site for converting excess carbohydrates and proteins into fatty acids and triglycerides, which are then transported and stored in fat tissue throughout the body. Glucose entering the blood after a meal is rapidly taken up by the liver and stored as large sugar molecules called glycogen through a process called glycogenesis. Later in the day, when blood concentrations of glucose begin to decline, the liver activates other pathways that allow this stored sugar to re-enter the blood for transport to all other tissues. This is needed as a survival mechanism during starvation or food shortage. When liver glycogen reserves become exhausted, which can occur when we have not eaten for several hours, the liver recognizes the problem and will activate an additional group of enzymes that begins synthesizing glucose out of such things as amino acids and stored fat reserves that increase our blood sugar for use as fuel. The ability of the liver to synthesize this "new"glucose is of supreme importance especially to carnivores, which have diets that are virtually devoid of starch.

3. Although the liver plays a role in so many aspects of human health, most of us recognize the liver's primary role in fat metabolism. The liver plays a part in most aspects of fat metabolism including the following.

Oxidation of triglycerides to produce energy. The liver breaks down many more fatty acids than the hepatocytes (liver cells) need, and transports large quantities of the surplus acetoacetate into the blood where it can be picked up and readily utilized by other tissues. The bulk of the lipoproteins such as cholesterol and phospholipids are synthesized in the liver. Some of these are packaged with lipoproteins and made available to the rest of the body. The remainder is excreted in bile as cholesterol or is converted to bile acids.

The liver activates and converts the B vitamins riboflavin, thiamine, pyridoxine, nicotinamide, pantothenic acid, and biotin into phosphate complexes that are more easily used in the body. It converts folic acid to folinic acid, vitamin B12 into its coenzyme forms, vitamin D into 25-hydroxy vitamin D and vitamin A into retinoic acid. The alterations of these vitamins by the liver are essential before they can perform their metabolic functions.

The liver is the largest gland in the body and a storage site for vitamins A, D, C, B12, riboflavin, pantothenic acid, folic acid, biotin, and pyridoxine. In the average person, the capacity for storage of vitamins A, D, and B12 can be large enough to last from six months to two years. Despite this capacity, deficiencies are still common. Vitamins A, B, C, D, and K are synthesized and transported in the liver. All other vitamins must be replenished from dietary or supplementary sources almost daily. The liver synthesizes inositol, choline, and lecithin. It converts cholesterol into bile salts (dependent on vitamin C) and produces proteins needed for blood clotting (dependent on vitamin K).

4. Perhaps one of the most important jobs the liver has is cleaning the blood through the removal or metabolizing of medications, hormones, and environmental and cellular toxins.

Toxins can be assimilated from the environment or created by our own system and reabsorbed through poor bowel function or a spastic bowel condition. Constipation or poor bowel function contributes considerably to systemic and liver toxicity, as does improper kidney function. If these organs of elimination don't function properly, or regularly, at least once per day, preferably after every meal for bowel function and several times a day for urinary function, then these same waste materials that should pass through our system daily can eventually end up in the blood due to a condition called permeable gut syndrome. The liver can successfully metabolize these extra toxins for a while, but eventually the liver will be overwhelmed.

Once in the liver, those toxic substances, are detoxified, metabolized, broken down, and eliminated via bile secretion. Many medications are removed from the bloodstream by the liver; but some use the liver to meter out the medication, which in turn ensures a constant amount entering the bloodstream.

The liver deactivates hormones, especially female hormones. It has estrogen receptors for this purpose, but when this role deteriorates, liver palm, spider mole, low libido, and male breast development are some of the possible long-term effects.

The liver produces important proteins that affect the blood, such as factors that are essential in making the blood clot after an injury. Proteins are made up of amino acids that need to be changed or joined together or changed in other ways to be used by the body. Synthesis of non-essential amino acids also occurs in the liver.

An important part of protein use is how the liver handles ammonia, the waste product of protein metabolism. Ammonia is changed into urea, the primary ingredient in urine, and excreted from the body by route of the kidneys, which filter urea out of the blood. Ammonia is very toxic and is easily absorbed by central nervous system tissues and if not rapidly and efficiently removed from circulation, it will result in injury to the central nervous system.

Other aspects of liver function include enzyme creation and activation needed for a host of biochemical processes throughout the body. The liver creates enzymes that convert proteins into sugars or lipids (fats). Several of the enzymes used in these pathways (for example, alanine and aspartate aminotransferases) are commonly used as measures of liver function in clinical blood tests.

Hepatocytes are responsible for synthesis of most plasma proteins. Albumin, a major plasma protein, is synthesized almost exclusively by the liver. Also, the liver synthesizes many of the clotting factors necessary for blood coagulation.

Due to these numerous and varied activities, the liver is exposed to a number of insults and is one of the organs most subject to injury. For this reason, the liver has one of the highest turnovers of cells in the body. It is because of this ability that it can replicate itself so quickly.

Threats to Liver Health

Poor Water Quality

Water safety cannot be taken for granted. As more chlorine is needed to maintain minimum safety standards for municipal water systems, this chemical will come to represent an increasingly greater threat to public health, including liver health.

In 1998, close to one thousand community drinking water supply systems, affecting about eighteen million people, violated EPA's Surface Water Treatment Rule, which was aimed at guarding against a micro-organism known as giardia and viruses in drinking-water supplies. About 7.9 million people were affected by violations of federal health standards for total coliform bacteria in 1998, which represents the vast majority of violations of federal health standards by community water systems. According to a recent audit of public water systems, 90 percent of monitoring and reporting violations, which should have been reported to the government, were reported incorrectly or not at all. Easy access to clean, safe water can no longer be taken for granted anywhere in the world, says a report by the American Academy of Microbiology. Growing populations, aging sewer systems, environmental pollution, and developing resistance of micro-organisms to water-treatment chemicals are among problems cited by the academy in its report "A Global Decline in Microbiological Safety of Water: A Call for Action," based on data from U.S. and international health agencies.

Poor Nutrition

Diet is one of the most important factors in maintaining overall liver health. We eat every day, so the daily food choices made will affect overall health dramatically. No single meal can dramatically change your health; rather it is the daily consumption of any food or drink that primarily affects the liver and the rest of your system. Just as there are certain foods and drinks that will create toxicity and liver damage there are foods and components of foods that are cleansing and healthy.

An example of this includes flavonoids and carotenoids, both vital components for health that have antiviral properties and are found in a wide range of foods. For example, flavanones are found in citrus, isoflavones in soy products, anthocyanidins in wine and bilberry, and flavans in apples and tea. Carotenoids are found in carrots and any other brightly colored vegetable such as sweet potatoes.

The U.S. Department of Agriculture initiated a nutritional study in 2000. During this study, the USDA monitored the food intake of twenty-one thousand people over three days, totaling almost two hundred thousand meals. It was reported that not one person of the twenty-one thousand involved received the minimum RDA of ten essential nutrients over the three days.

This discovery is troubling, but even more disquieting is the fact that the RDA is the barest minimum that we need in order to maintain bodily function without lapsing into a chronic deficiency state. Despite this, in the general population, the vast majority of us cannot even maintain this minimal level of nutrition. It is no wonder that the incidence of chronic disease such as cancer and arthritis and general ill health are rising every year. The major reason for the majority of these conditions is malnutrition or nutrient deficiency. The question we need to ask ourselves is not whether we need to supplement our diet, but rather, "What kind, how much, and how often do I need to take supplements to maintain good health?" Along with this question we must ask ourselves, "What can I do to get the most out of the supplements I use?"

Pollution

While many of us have to live with polluted air, we can reduce its effects by the choices we make daily in diet and supplements, water quality and quantity, and systemic cleansing. Much of the pollution we are subjected to has a cumulative effect. Cleansing the liver and the rest of the eliminatory system will reduce this buildup. This practice should be repeated on a regular basis in order to keep up with the constant exposure to pollutants.

Alcohol

Alcoholic cirrhosis is one of the major causes of liver damage. More than two million people currently have alcoholic cirrhosis in the United States. That's one in 136 people. In 1999, almost twelve thousand deaths from cirrhosis and other conditions directly related to alcohol were reported.

Some drinkers develop alcoholic hepatitis or inflammation of the liver as a result of long-term heavy drinking. Its symptoms include fever, jaundice, and abdominal pain. Alcoholic hepatitis can cause death if drinking continues.

Drug Use

Both illicit drugs and prescription drugs have a real potential to create liver problems even after a short period of use. With illicit drugs, especially with injectable drugs, there is the added risk of contracting AIDS or hepatitis from infected needles. Talk to your doctor about the likelihood of liver damage from any prescriptions you use.

Disease

Infectious disease can create liver damage as well. For infectious (viral) hepatitis, good hygiene is necessary to avoid spreading the infection. The hepatitis A virus can be spread very easily through food that is handled by infected individuals; therefore, people with hepatitis A should wash their hands very carefully after using the restroom and should not handle food at work. The hepatitis viruses B and C are both transmitted by blood and sexual contact.

Stress

High stress is now known to play a role in liver health. Most of us can't reduce our stress, but we can still reduce the effect on our liver from long-term stress by cleansing and eating a good diet along with supplements and exercise.

The Liver's Amazing Powers of Regeneration

The liver's hepatocytes have a unique capacity to reproduce in response to liver injury. An example of liver regeneration occurs after surgical removal of a portion of the liver or after an injury that destroys part of the liver. In fact, this property plays a major role in modern liver transplant operations. The liver has a remarkable capacity to regenerate after injury and to adjust its size to match its host. Within a week after partial removal of the liver (hepatectomy), which in typical experimental settings entails surgical removal of two-thirds of the liver, the donor liver's size returns to its pre-surgical size.

Some additional interesting observations include: In the few cases where baboon livers have been transplanted into people, they quickly grow to the size of a human liver. When the liver from a large dog is transplanted into a small dog, it loses mass until it reaches the size appropriate for a small dog, with the reverse also being true.

Hepatocytes (liver cells) transplanted to other areas of the body remain dormant but begin to grow in number after partial hepatectomy (surgical reduction of the liver) of the host. Amazingly, these cells that are separated from the liver mass still know when more liver function is needed and increase in number automatically no matter where they are situated in the body.

Liver Cleansing

We've all heard the phrase "an ounce of prevention is worth a pound of cure." Nowhere is this more appropriate than in maintaining optimal liver health through regular cleansing.

The liver processes nutrients found in food and neutralizes environmental poisons. Did you know that abnormal liver test results typically become evident only after 50 percent of the liver has been damaged? Doesn't it make sense to take preventive action rather than wait until blood tests show abnormal functioning of this most important organ? Many people use supplements in an effort to improve health and slow down the aging process, and this is a wonderful first step on the journey towards improved health and longevity.

Even modern medical research is interested in the association between environmental toxins and chronic disease. It has been estimated that between five hundred billion and eight hundred billion dollars are spent annually in North America in treating toxicity-related chronic disease.

It is theorized that environmental contaminants are causative factors in the emergence of several chronic conditions, including Parkinson's disease, several types of cancers, chronic fatigue syndrome, and possibly diabetes and atherosclerosis.

Environmental toxins and contaminants may account for almost 80 percent of all cancer cases, which is particularly upsetting considering that cancer is the third most common cause of death for children.

Due to children's increased exposure to organochlorinated pesticides between 1973 and 1997, two particular cancers, non-Hodgkin's lymphoma and brain cancer, have increased in children by 30 percent and 21 percent respectively.

As the liver becomes slowly more toxic over the years from both internal and environmental pollution and poisons, changes start to occur that at first are subtle but become more persistent and debilitating as time goes on.

According to the U.S. National Center for Health Statistics, the tenth most frequent cause of death among males is liver cancer and related conditions, with too many men dying prematurely from a condition that may be prevented by doing regular liver cleanses.

Herbs and Supplements for Liver Cleansing

Healers have long used plants to prevent and cure illness. Several cultures, such as Chinese, Indian, and Native American, have developed their own traditions, practices, and usages that are passed from generation to generation.

Some of the herbs profiled here, such as peony and bupleurum, are usually used in traditional Chinese medicine. The system of herbal medicine that developed in China differs in several significant ways from European herbal medicine.

One of the more obvious differences between Western and

Chinese herbalism is that Western herbalists often concentrate on treating illness with a single herb; in traditional Chinese medicine, herbalists typically use herbs in combinations called formulas and practice preventive medicine by treating the patient before illness occurs. Traditional Chinese formulas are specific to each individual and are compounded in strict accordance with the patient's constitution according to the complex principles of traditional Chinese medicine.

Milk Thistle (*Silybum marianum*)

Native to Europe, milk thistle has a long history of use as food and medicine in folklore. Milk thistle has been used as a remedy since ancient Greece, where the herbalist Dioscorides used it to treat snakebites. As a result of its long history in human use and research conducted by German researchers in the 1960s, Germany's Commission E approved an oral extract of milk thistle in 1986 for treatment of liver disease.

Common Uses

Alcoholic cirrhosis, viral hepatitis, cirrhosis, liver toxicity, and damage due to drug and chemical exposure, and ingestion of death cap mushroom (*Amanita phalloides*).

Constituents

When dried, the fruit of the milk thistle contains 1 percent to 4 percent of four isomers (polyphenolic flavanolignins) called collectively silymarin. They consist of silybin or silibinin, isosilibin, silydianin, and silycristin.

Milk thistle also contains flavonoids, betaine, trimethylglycine, and amines. Silibinin is the most biologically active of the four polyphenolic flavanolignins. Silycristin is a metabolic stimulant, and silibinin is the most hepatoprotective.

Scientific Research/Validation

Animal studies have shown that milk thistle extracts to be of value in toxicity caused by chemicals such as polycyclic aromatic hydrocarbons, acetaminophen, carbon tetrachloride, and ethanol.

Human studies have had similar results. A Hungarian study reported that thirty workers suffering from long-term exposure to toluene and other organic solvents showed significant improvement in liver enzymes after a thirty-day treatment with milk thistle.

Studies of chronic and acute viral hepatitis found significant improvements in symptoms such as fatigue and abdominal pain and improved liver enzyme test results after treatment with milk thistle. However, a recent multi-center study involving two hundred patients with alcoholic cirrhosis failed to show statistically significant effectiveness of silymarin in changing the course of the disease in groups studied. But one Austrian study reported a 58 percent survival rate after four years for patients using milk thistle extract for two years. In comparison, there was only a 39 percent survival rate in the placebo group.

In several similar human double-blind, placebo-controlled studies, milk thistle improved overall liver function in a group of alcoholic cirrhosis patients after only four weeks of treatment. Milk thistle increases RNA activity and protein synthesis in rats, which may explain the tissue regeneration effects of milk thistle.

Toxicity

Despite being widely used in Europe since 1969, no adverse events have been reported even after long-term use of milk thistle. Animal studies have also reported very low levels of toxicity.

Drug Interactions

Milk thistle may reduce the hepatotoxicity of many minerals, drugs, and chemicals including: Acetaminophen, Phenothiazines, Cisplatin, Cyclosporin, Ethanol, Aspirin, Halothane, carbon tetrachloride, iron, and Dilantin.

A potential added benefit is that milk thistle very well could increase the effectiveness of the drugs Cisplatin and Doxorubicin, which are two of the most commonly used drugs to treat uterine, vaginal, ovarian, and breast cancer.

SAMe (S-adenosylmethionine)

SAMe is a relative newcomer to the nutritional supplement scene, but it has proven to be valuable in treating several conditions and it is considered to be essential in over forty different physiological processes.

Common Uses

One important property of SAMe is its ability to increase bile flow even in damaged livers. This is especially important in the treatment of diseases such as Gilbert's Syndrome, cirrhosis, cholestasis, and alcoholic liver injury.

In cirrhosis, one outcome is that formation of SAMe from metabolism of methionine is prevented. As a result, one study reported a 47 percent lower rate of death and need for liver transplant in chronic alcoholics with cirrhosis with the administration of a long-term (two-year) dosage of SAMe.

The effect of SAMe is even more pronounced in less severe cases of cirrhosis; the earlier you start using SAMe, the better the results will be.

Dandelion (*Taraxacum officinale*)

Closely related to chicory, dandelion is a common plant worldwide and the mortal enemy of those who love a perfect lawn. Dandelion is grown commercially in the United States and Europe, and the leaves and roots are used in numerous herbal supplements.

Common Uses

Dandelion in the past was commonly used as a food with the leaves being used in salads and teas, while the baked roots were sometimes used as a coffee substitute.

Dandelion leaves and roots have been used for hundreds of

years to treat kidney ailments leading to water retention, liver conditions and gallbladder and joint problems. In addition, it has been used to treat eczema and cancer and to cleanse the blood.

Constituents

The primary constituents responsible for dandelion's action on the digestive system and liver are the bitter principles or chemicals. Previously referred to as taraxacin, these constituents are sesquiterpene lactones of the eudesmanolide and germacranolide type, and are unique to dandelion. Dandelion is also a rich source of vitamins and minerals. The leaves have a high content of vitamin A as well as moderate amounts of vitamin D, vitamin C, various B vitamins, iron, silicon, magnesium, zinc, and manganese.

Scientific Research/Validation

An animal study reported that dandelion leaves can be as effective as the diuretic drug furosemide if the dose is great enough (2 grams per 2.2 pounds of body weight). Unfortunately, current human studies have not corroborated the results of these animal trials.

As water retention can be a sign of a more serious disorder of the kidneys, it is recommended that individuals wishing to use dandelion as a part of their treatment check this possibility out with their doctor. Dandelion not only helps in edema but has traditionally been used to accelerate digestion and bowel function while increasing bile production and secretion from the liver and gallbladder

Toxicity

Dandelion leaves and roots should not be used by people with gallstones or with any bile-duct obstruction without the supervision of a physician.

Dandelion has been reported to stimulate an overabundance of stomach acid, which should be avoided by anyone with gastric ulcers. Some individuals may experience an allergic rash reaction to the latex found in the stem and leaves of dandelion.

Phyllanthus (*Phyllanthus niruri*)

This herb has been a mainstay in ayurvedic medicine for several thousand years and is indigenous to southern and central India. Other members of the same family are grown in China, Cuba, Nigeria, Guam, and the Philippines.

Common Uses

Phyllanthus has been used in ayurvedic medicine for over two thousand years and has a wide number of traditional uses. It has been used for skin conditions such as ulcers, bedsores, swelling, and itchiness. Internal uses include treatment for heavy or frequent periods, jaundice, diabetes, and gonorrhea.

Constituents

Phyllanthus primarily contains lignans (e.g., phyllanthine and hypophyllanthine), alkaloids, and flavonoids (e.g., quercetin). One constituent stops the production of the critical enzyme DNA polymerase that hepatitis B needs to replicate.

Scientific Research/Validation

Research has proven that phyllanthus will improve or eradicate one of the blood markers associated with hepatitis B in 59 percent of all cases with a dose of 900 mg used for only thirty days. Several species are used, however *P. urinaria* and *P. niruri* work more effectively than *P. amarus*. A typical dose would be 900–2,700 mg daily.

Toxicity

No known side effects or drug reactions have been reported.

Bupleurum (*Bupleurum chinense, Bupleurum falcatum*)

Common Uses

Bupleurum has been a major herb used in traditional Chinese medicine for millennia primarily for the treatment of liver conditions, fever, hemorrhoids, indigestion, and prolapse of the uterus. Bupleurum makes up 16 percent of the formula for *sho-saiko-to*, a classic liver formula used for centuries.

Constituents

Saikosaponins have the foremost biological activity with in vitro studies that reportedly prove that cytokine production is markedly increased, resulting in increased immune cell communication.

These same saponins also reduce the growth of liver cancer cells and inflammation.

Scientific Research/ Validation

To date, only one human double-blind study has reported that the sho-saiko-to formula containing bupleurum can help reduce blood liver enzymes and other symptoms in individuals with active viral hepatitis.

While most of these studies have been conducted on patients with hepatitis B, one hepatitis C trial published similar positive findings. An unblinded study reported sho-saiko-to reduced liver cancer rates in cirrhosis and hepatitis patients.

Peony (*Paeonia suffruticosa, Paeonia lactiflora, Paeonia veitchii*)

Common Uses

Three similar plants are all called peony, and different parts are used in different cases. The bark of the root of *Paeonia suffruticosa* is called *moutan* or *mu dan* in China, where it naturally grows. Red peony root comes from wild harvested *Paeonia lactiflora* or *Paeonia veitchii*. White peony root comes from cultivated *Paeonia lactiflora*. The bark, red peony root, and white peony root all have somewhat different properties. Dried versus charred roots also have different properties. The color indicated does not refer to flower color. An important formula used in Chinese and Japanese herbal medicine called *shakuyaku-kanzo-to* contains white peony root and licorice root. The roots and flowers of *Paeonia officinalis* have been used in European herbal medicine. However, the German Commission E did not approve this plant for medicinal use.

Constituents

Peony contains a unique glycoside called paeoniflorin. Proanthocyanidins, flavonoids, tannins, polysaccharides, and paeoniflorin are all considered to contribute to the medicinal activity of various forms of peony. Paeoniflorin's major effect seems to be to calm nerves and alleviate spasms. One study has confirmed the efficacy of shakuyaku-kanzo-to (formula with peony and licorice) for relieving muscle cramps due to cirrhosis of the liver, diabetes, and dialysis.

Scientific Research/Validation

Shakuyaku-kanzo-to is approved by the Japanese Ministry of Health and Welfare for treatment of muscle cramps. Another Japanese formulation known as *toki-shakuyaku-san* combines peony root with dong quai and four other herbs and has been found to effectively reduce symptoms of cramping and pain associated with dysmenorrhea (painful menses). Paeoniflorin and peony extracts also enhance mental function in animal studies, suggesting a potential benefit for dementia. Human studies have not yet been conducted to confirm this theory. Red peony root and moutan bark have both shown antioxidant activity in vitro, likely due to the presence of paeoniflorin, proanthocyanidins, and flavonoids. Polysaccharides found in peony bark and root have shown an ability to stimulate immune cells in the test tube. Animal studies have found that red peony root, alone or in combination with other Chinese herbs, could help prevent liver damage due to various chemical toxins. A crude extract of red peony root was shown in a small preliminary trial to reduce liver fibrosis in some patients with chronic viral hepatitis. Other case studies published in Chinese have found red peony root helpful for people with viral hepatitis. Crude red peony root extracts and combinations of these extracts with other Chinese herbs inhibit platelet aggregation, thrombosis, and excessive clotting in vitro and in vivo. A rabbit study found that peony was effective at lowering cholesterol levels in the aorta.

Ornithine (L-ornithine-L-aspartate, OA, Ornithine-aspartate)

Ornithine, an amino acid, is manufactured by the body when another amino acid, arginine, is metabolized during the production of urea (a constituent of urine).

Scientific Research/Validation

Ornithine aspartate has been shown to be beneficial in people with brain abnormalities (hepatic encephalopathy) due to liver cirrhosis. In a double-blind trial, people with cirrhosis and hepatic encephalopathy received either 18 grams per day of L-ornithine-L-aspartate or a placebo for two weeks. Those taking the ornithine had significant improvements in liver function and blood tests compared with those taking the placebo.

Toxicity

No side effects have been reported with the use of ornithine, except for gastrointestinal distress with intakes over 10 grams per day. The presence of arginine is needed to produce ornithine in the body, so higher levels of this amino acid should increase ornithine production. There are currently no known drug interactions with ornithine.

Betaine (Trimethylglycine)
Common Uses

Betaine (trimethylglycine) functions very closely with choline, folic acid, vitamin B12, and a form of the amino acid methionine known as S-adenosylmethionine (SAMe). All of these compounds function as "methyl donors." They carry and donate methyl molecules to facilitate necessary chemical processes. The donation of methyl groups by betaine is very important to proper liver function, cellular replication, and detoxification. Betaine also plays a role in the manufacture of carnitine and serves to protect the kidneys from damage. Betaine is closely related to choline. The difference is that choline (tetramethylglycine) has four methyl groups attached to it. When choline donates one of these groups to another molecule, it becomes betaine (trimethylglycine). If betaine donates one of its methyl groups, then it becomes dimethylglycine.

Scientific Research/Validation

Betaine is often referred to as a lipotropic factor because of its ability to help the liver process lipids. In animal studies, betaine supplementation has been shown to protect against chemical damage to the liver. The first stage of liver damage that results from drinking alcohol is the accumulation of fat in the liver (alcohol-induced fatty liver disease). Betaine, because of its lipotropic effects, has been shown to produce significant improvements in this condition in several human clinical studies. Betaine has been studied in clinical trials conducted in Germany, Italy, and France in the treatment of alcohol-related liver disease. Some success was noted in these studies, but the popularity of betaine for alcohol-related liver disease has been supplanted by SAMe and milk thistle extract. However, it has recently been suggested that betaine may be a more cost-effective method as a first-step therapy for alcohol-induced fatty liver disease.

Toxicity

No side effects or drug interactions from using betaine at recommended levels have been reported.

Methionine

Methionine is one of the essential amino acids (building blocks of protein), meaning that it cannot be produced by the body, and must be provided in the diet. It supplies sulfur and other compounds required by the body for normal metabolism and growth. Methionine also belongs to a group of compounds called lipotropics, or chemicals that help the liver process fats (lipids). Others in this group include choline, inositol, and betaine.

Toxicity

Animal studies suggest that diets high in methionine in the presence of B-vitamin deficiencies may increase the risk for atherosclerosis by increasing blood levels of cholesterol and homocysteine. This idea has not yet been tested in humans. Excessive methionine intake, together with an inadequate intake of folic acid, vitamin B6, and vitamin B12, can increase the conversion of methionine to homocysteine—a substance linked to heart disease and stroke. Even in the absence of a deficiency of folic acid, B6, or B12, megadoses of methionine (7 grams per day) have been found to cause elevations in blood levels of homocysteine. Whether such an increase would create a significant hazard for humans taking supplemental methionine has not been established. Supplementation of up to 2 grams of methionine daily for long periods of time has not been reported to cause any serious side effects.

Branched-Chain Amino Acids (BCAAs, Isoleucine, Leucine, Valine)

Branched-chain amino acids are considered essential amino acids because humans cannot survive unless these amino acids are present in the diet. BCAAs are needed for the maintenance of muscle tissue and appear to preserve muscle stores of glycogen (a carbohydrate that can be converted into energy). BCAAs also help prevent muscle protein breakdown during exercise.

Scientific Research/Validation

Patients with liver diseases that lead to coma, such as hepatic encephalopathy, have low concentrations of BCAAs and excess levels of certain other amino acids. Preliminary research suggests that people with this condition might be helped by BCAAs. Double-blind studies have produced somewhat inconsistent results, but a re-analysis of these studies found an overall benefit for the treatment of encephalopathy. Therapeutic effects of BCAAs have also been shown in children with liver failure and adults with cirrhosis. Treatment of liver failure requires immediate emergency medical intervention.

Aging Well

Due to the baby boom, there will soon be more people over the age of sixty in North America than at any other time in history. This is particularly relevant to liver health. Until recently, liver damage was almost nonexistent in younger people, but even this statistic is changing. Prior to the 1950s, liver ailments did not usually begin to manifest until age forty due to toxin accumulation and neglect over time. As the use of chemicals increases in our food chain and throughout the environment, liver problems begin to manifest in younger segments of the population. To ensure that we age well and remain healthy, it becomes a priority to maintain proper liver function.

References

Adverse Drug Reactions Advisory Committee. An adverse reaction to the herbal medication milk thistle [Silybum marianum]. *Med J Aust* 1999: 170: 218–9.

Angelico M, Gandin C, Nistri A, et al. Oral S-adenosyl-L-methionine (SAMe) administration enhances bile salt conjugation with taurine in patients with liver cirrhosis. *Scand J Clin Lab Invest* 1994; 54: 459–64.

Awang D. Milk thistle. *Can Pharm J* 1993; 422; 403–4.

Babucke G, Sarre B. Clinical experience with betain citrate. *Med Klin* 1973; 68: 1109–13 [in German].

Barak AJ, Beckenhauer HC, Badakhsh S, Tuma DJ. The effect of betaine in reversing alcoholic steatosis. *Alcohol Clin Exp Res* 1997; 21: 1100–2.

Barak AJ, Beckenhauer HC, Matti J, Tuma DJ. Dietary betaine promotes generation of hepatic S-adenosylmethioine and protects the liver from ethanol-induced fatty infiltration. *Alcohol Clin Exp Res* 1993; 17: 552–5.

Barak AJ, Beckenhauer HC, Tuma DJ. Betaine, ethanol, and the liver: a review. *Alcohol* 1996; 13: 395–8 [review].

Barak AJ, Tuma DJ. Betaine, metabolic by-product or vital methylating agent? *Life Sci* 1983; 32: 771–4 [review].

Bensky D, Gamble A, Kaptchuk T. *Chinese Herbal Medicine Materia Medica*, rev ed. Seattle: Eastland Press, 1993, 49–50.

Berenguer J, Carrasco D. Double-blind trial of silymarin vs. placebo in the treatment of chronic hepatitis. *Munch Med Wochenschr.* 1977; 119: 240–260.

Bharatiya VB. *Selected Medicinal Plants of India*. Bombay: Tata Press, 1992, 235–7.

Blomstrand E, Ek S, Newsholme EA. Influence of ingesting a solution of branched-chain amino acids on plasma and muscle concentrations of amino acids during prolonged submaximal exercise. *Nutrition* 1996; 12: 485–90.

Blumenthal M, Busse WR, Goldberg A, et al. (eds). *The Complete Commission E Monographs: Therapeutic Guide to Herbal Medicines*. Boston, MA: Integrative Medicine Communications, 1998, 118–20.

Böhm K. Choleretic action of some medicinal plants. *Arzneimittelforschung* 1959; 9: 376–8.

Bombardieri G, Milani A, Bernardi L, Rossi L. Effects of S-adenosyl-L-methionine (SAMe) in the treatment of Gilbert's syndrome. *Curr Ther Res* 1985; 37: 580–5.

Bradley PR (ed). *British Herbal Compendium*, Vol 1. Bournemouth, Dorset, UK: British Herbal Medicine Association, 1992, 73–5.

Buckley JD, Meadows AT, Kadin ME, Le Beau MM, Siegel S, Robison LL. Pesticide exposures in children with non-Hodgkin's lymphoma. Cancer. 2000; 89(11): 2315–21.

Buzzelli G, Moscarella S, Giusti A, et al. A pilot study on the liver-protective effect of silybin-phosphatidylcholine complex (IdB 1016) in chronic active hepatitis. Int J Clin Pharmacol Ther Toxicol. 1993; 31: 456–460.

Cachin M, Pergola F. Betaine aspartate in the hepato-digestive domain. Sem Ther 1966; 42: 423–4 [in French].

Cairella M, Volpari B. Betaine aspartate in the therapy of liver diseases. Clin Ter 1972; 60: 513-34 [in Italian].

CDC. National Center for Health Statistics. 2000.; NCI. SEER Cancer Statistics Review, 1973-1997.

Chambers ST. Betaines: their significance for bacteria and the renal tract. Clin Sci 1995; 88: 25-7 [review].

Chin SE, Sheperd RW, Thomas BJ, et al. Nutritional support in children with end-stage liver disease: a randomized crossover trial of a branched-chain amino acid supplement. Am J Clin Nutr 1992; 56: 158-63.

Daniels JL, Olshan AF, Savitz DA. Pesticides and childhood cancers. Environ Health Perspect. 1997; 105(10): 1068-77.

Egberts E-H, et al. Branched chain amino acids in the treatment of latent portosystemic encephalopathy. Gastroenterology 1985; 88: 887-95.

Feher J, Desk G, Muzes G, et al. Liver protective action of silymarin therapy in chronic alcoholic liver diseases [in Hungarian]. Orv Hetil. 1989; 130: 2723–2727.

Ferenci P, Dragosics B, Dittrich H, Frank H, Benda L, Lochs H, Meryn S, Base W, Schneider B. Randomized controlled trial of silymarin treatment in patients with cirrhosis of the liver. 1st Department of Gastroenterology and Hepatology, University of Vienna, Austria. J Hepatol 1989 Jul; 9(1): 105-13.

Flora K, Hahn M, Rosen H, et al. Milk thistle (Silybum marianum) for the therapy of liver disease. Am Gastroenterol 1998; 93: 139-43.

Foster S, Yue CX. Herbal Emissaries: Bringing Chinese Herbs to the West. Rochester, VT: Healing Arts Press, 1992: 200–7.

Frezza M, Surrenti C, Manzillo G, et al. Oral S-adenosyl-methionine in the symptomatic treatment of intrahepatic cholestasis: a double-blind, placebo-controlled study. Gastroenterology 1990; 99: 211–5.

Fujiwara K, Ohta Y, Ogata I, et al. Treatment trial of traditional Oriental medicine in chronic viral hepatitis. In: Ohta Y (ed). New Trends in Peptic Ulcer and Chronic Hepatitis: Part II. Chronic Hepatitis. Tokyo: Excerpta Medica, 1987, 141–6.

Gaedeke J, Fels LM, Bokemeyer C, et al. Cisplatin nephrotoxicity and protection by silybinin. Nephro Dial Transplant 1996; 11: 55-62.

Gibo Y, Nakamura Y, Takahashi N, et al. Clinical study of sho-saiko-to therapy for Japanese patients with chronic hepatitis C (CH-C). Prog Med 1994; 14: 217–9.

Hilt G, Tuzin P. Clinical results using betaine citrate (Flacar) in fatty livers. Med Monatsschr 1973; 27: 322-5 [in German].

Hilt G, Tuzin P. Clinical results using betaine citrate (Flacar) in fatty livers. Med Monatsschr 1973; 27: 322-5 [in German].

Hirayama C, Okumura M, Tanikawa K, et al. A multicenter randomized controlled clinical trial of sho-saiko-to in chronic active hepatitis. *Gastroent Jap* 1989; 24: 715–9.

Junnila M, Barak AJ, Beckenhauer HC, Rahko T. Betaine reduces hepatic lipidosis induced by carbon tetrachloride in Sprague-Dawley rats. *Vet Hum Toxicol* 1998; 40: 263-6.

Kandziora J. Therapeutic experience with the lipotropic hepatic drug Flacar in the internal medicine practice. *ZFA* 1976; 52: 1561-3 [in German].

Kato M, Miwa Y, Tajika M, et al. Preferential use of branched-chain amino acids as an energy substrate in patients with liver cirrhosis. *Intern Med* 1998; 37: 429-34.

Kim SK, Kim YC, Kim YC. Effects of singly administered betaine on hepatotoxicity of chloroform in mice. *Food Chem Toxicol* 1998; 36: 655-61.

Kotani N, Oyama T, Hashimoto H, et al. Analgesic effect of a herbal medicine for treatment of primary dysmenorrhea—a double-blind study. *Am J Chin Med* 1997; 25: 205–12.

Kuusi T, Pyylaso H, Autio K. The bitterness properties of dandelion. II. Chemical investigations. *Lebensm-Wiss Technol* 1985; 18: 347–9.

Leach FN, Braganza JM. Methionine is important in treatment of chronic pancreatitis. *Br Med J* 1998; 316: 474 [letter].

Lichtenstein P, Holm NV, Verkasalo PK, et al. Environmental and heritable factors in the causation of cancer. N Eng J Med. 2000; 343: 78-85.

Lieber CS. Herman Award lecture, 1993: a personal perspective on alcohol, nutrition, and the liver. *Am J Clin Nutr* 1993; 58: 430–42 [review].

Lirussi F, Okolicsanyi L. Cytoprotection in the nineties: Experience with ursodeoxycholic acid and silymarin in chronic liver disease. Acta Physiol Hung. 1992; 80: 363–367.

Luper S. A review of plants used in the treatment of liver disease: part l. Altem Med Rev 1998; 3: 410-21.

MacLean DA, Graham TE, Saltin B. Branched-chain amino acids augment ammonia metabolism while attenuating protein breakdown during exercise. *Am J Physiol* 1994; 267: E1010-22.

Maddrey WC. Branched chain amino acid therapy in liver disease. *J Am Coll Nutr* 1985; 4: 639-50 [review].

Mato JM, Cámara J, Fernández J, et al. S-adenosylmethionine in alcoholic liver cirrhosis: a randomized, placebo-controlled, double-blind, multicenter clinical trial. J Hepatol 1999; 30: 1081–9.

McAuley DF, Hanratty CG, McGurk C, et al. Effect of methionine supplementation on endothelial function, plasma homocysteine, and lipid peroxidation. *J Toxicol Clin Toxicol* 1999; 37: 435–40.

Meinert R, Schuz J, Kaletsch U, Kaatsch P, Michaelis J. Leukemia and non-Hodgkin's lymphoma in childhood and exposure to pesticides: results of a register-based case-control study in Germany. Am J Epidemiol. 2000; 151(7): 639-46, 647-50.

Meixa W, Haowei C, Yanjun L, et al. Herbs of the genus *Phyllanthus* in the treatment of chronic hepatitis B: observation with three preparations from different geographic sites. *J Lab Clin Med* 1995; 126: 350–2.

Motoo Y, Sawabu N. Antitumor effects of saikosaponins, baicalin and baicalein on human hepatoma cell lines. *Cancer Lett* 1994; 86: 91–5.

Muir T, Zegarac M. Societal costs of exposure to toxic substances: economic and health costs of four case studies that are candidates for environmental causation. Environ Health Perspect. 2001; 109 Suppl 6: 885-903.

Murakami T, Nagamura Y, Hirano K. The recovering effect of betaine on carbon tetrachloride-induced liver injury. *J Nutr Sci Vitaminol* 1998; 44: 249-55.

Muriel P, Garciapina T, Perez-Alvarcz V, et al. Silymarin protects against Paracetamol-induced lipid peroxidation and liver damage. J Appi Toxicol 1992; 12: 439-42.

Muriel P, Mourelle M. Prevention by silymarin of membrane alterations in acute CCL liver damage, J Appi Toxicol 1990; 10: 275-9.

Murray MT. Milk thistle. In: The healing power of herbs. 2nd ed. Rocklin (CA): Prima Publishing; 1995. p. 243-51.

Nadkarmi KM. *India Materia Medica,* vol 1. Bombay: Popular Prakashan Private Ltd., 1993, 947–8.

Naylor CD, O'Rourke K, Detsky AS, et al. Parenteral nutrition with branched-chain amino acids in hepatic encephalopathy. A meta-analysis. *Gastroenterology* 1989; 97: 1033-42.

Nicrosini F. Therapeutic activity of betaine aspartate. *Clin Ter* 1972; 15; 61: 227-36 [in Italian].

Ohta H, Ni JW, Matsumoto K, et al. Paeony and its major constituent, paeoniflorin, improve radial maze performance impaired by scopolamine in rats. *Pharmacol Biochem Behav* 1993; 45: 719–23.

Oka H, Yamamoto S, Kuroki T, et al. Prospective study of chemoprevention of hepatocellular carcinoma with sho-saiko-to (TJ-9). *Cancer* 1995; 76: 743–9.

Okubo T, Nagai F, Seto T, et al. The inhibition of phenylhydroquinone-induced oxidative DNA cleavage by constituents of Moutan Cortex and Paeoniae Radix. *Biol Pharm Bull* 2000; 23: 199–203.

Olmstead MJ. Heavy metal sources, effects, and detoxification. Altern Ther Complement Med. 2000; Dec; 347-354.

Osman E, Owen JS, Burroughs AK. S-adenosyl-L-methionine–a new therapeutic agent in liver disease? Aliment Pharmacol Ther 1993; 7: 21–8 [review].

Pares A, Planas R, Torres M, et al. Effects of silymarin in alcoholic patients with cirrhosis of the liver: Results of a controlled, double blind, randomized and multicenter trial. Hepatol 1998; 28: 615-21.

Pietrangelo A, Borella F, Casalgrandi G, et al. Antioxidant activity of Silymarin in vivo during long term iron overload in rats. Gastroenterology 1995; 109: 1941-9.

Qi XG. Protective mechanism of *Salvia miltiorrhiza* and *Paeonia lactiflora* for experimental liver damage. *Chung Hsi I Chieh Ho Tsa Chih* 1991; 11: 69, 102–4 [in Chinese].

Racciatti D, Vecchiet J, Ceccomancini A, Ricci F, Pizzigallo E. Chronic fatigue syndrome following a toxic exposure. Sci Total Environ. 2001; 270(1-3): 27-31.

Racz-Kotilla E, Racz G, Solomon A. The action of *Taraxacum officinale* extracts on body weight and diuresis of laboratory animals. *Planta Med* 1974: 26: 212–7.

Salmi HA, Sarna S. Effect of silymarin on chemical, functional and morphological alterations of the liver. A double blind controlled study. Scand J Gastroenterol. 1982; 17: 517–521.

Scambia G, De Vincenzo R, Ranelletri FO, et al. Antiproliferative effect of silybin on gynaecological malignancies: synergism with cisplatin and doxorubicin. Eur J Cancer 1996; 32A: 877-82.

Schonfeld JV, Weisbrod B, Muller MK. Silybum, a plant extract with antioxidant and membrane stabilizing properties, protects exocrine pancreas from cyclosporin A toxicity. Cell Mol Life Sci 1997; 53: 917-20.

Selhub J. Homocysteine metabolism. *Annu Rev Nutr* 1999; 19: 217-46 [review].

Semmler F. Treatment of liver diseases, especially of fatty liver with betaine citrate. *Ther Ggw* 1977; 116: 2113-24 [in German].

Sherer TB, Betarbet R, Greenamyre JT. Environment, mitochondria, and Parkinson's disease. Neuroscientist. 2002; 8(3): 192-7.

Silkworth JB, Brown JF Jr. Evaluating the impact of exposure to environmental contaminants on human health. Clin Chem. 1996; 42: 8(B): 1345-49.

Sonnenbichler J, Scalera F, Sonnenbichler I, et al. Stimulatory effects of silibinin and silicristin from the milk thistle Silybum marianum on kidney cells. J Pharmacol Exp Ther 1999; 290: 1375-83.

Sonnenbichler J, Sonnenbichler I, Scalera F. Influence of the flavonolignan silibinin of milk thistle on hepatocytes and kidney cells. In: Lawson LD, Bauer R, editors. Phytomedicines of Europe: chemistry and biological activity. Washington: American Chemical Society; 1998. p. 263-77.

Stauch S, Kircheis G, Adler G, et al. Oral L-ornithine-L-aspartate therapy of chronic hepatic encephalopathy: results of a placebo-controlled double-blind study. *J Hepatol* 1998; 28: 856–64.

Szilard S, Szentgyorgyi D, Demeter I. Protective effect of Legalon in workers exposed to organic solvents. Tisza Chemical Works Leninvaros, Occupational Health Care Service, Hungary. Acta Med Hung 1988; 45(2): 249-56

Tajiri H, Kozaiwa K, Osaki Y, et al. The study of the effect of sho-saiko-to on HBeAg clearance in children with chronic HBV infection and with abnormal liver function tests. *Acta Paediatr Jpn* 1991; 94: 1811–5.

Tanasescu C, Petrea S, Baldescu R, Macarie E, Chiriloiu C, Purice S. Use of the Romanian product Silimarina in the treatment of chronic liver diseases. N. Gh. Lupu Institute of Internal Medicine, Bucharest, Romania. Med Interne 1988 Oct-Dec; 26(4): 311-22

Thyagarajan SP, Subramanian S, Thirunalasundar T, et al. Effect of *Phyllanthus amarus* on chronic carriers of hepatitis B virus. *Lancet* 1988: 2: 1017–8.

Toborek M, Hennig B. Is methionine an atherogenic amino acid? *J Optimal Nutr* 1994; 3: 80–3.

Tomoda M, Matsumoto K, Shimizu N, et al. An acidic polysaccharide with immunological activities from the root of *Paeonia lactiflora*. *Biol Pharm Bull* 1994; 17: 1161–4.

Tomoda M, Matsumoto K, Shimizu N, et al. Characterization of a neutral and an acidic polysaccharide having immunological activities from the root of *Paeonia lactiflora*. *Biol Pharm Bull* 1993; 16: 1207–10.

Utrilla MP, Zarzuelo A, Risco S, et al. Isolation of a saikosaponin responsible for the anti-inflammatory activity of *Bupleurum gibralticum* Lam root extract. *Phytother Res* 1991; 5: 43–5.

Valenzuela A, Lagos C, Schmidt K, et al. Silymarin protection against lipid peroxidation induced by acute ethanol intoxication in the rat. *Biochem Pharmacol* 1985; 34: 2209-12.

Vogel G, Tuchweber B, Trost W, et al. Protection by Silymarin against Amanita phalloides intoxication in beagles. *Toxicol Appi Pharmacol* 1984; 73: 355-62.

Wagner H. Antihepatotoxic flavonoids. In: Cody V, Middleton E Jr, Hardborne JB, editors. Plant flavonoids in biology and medicine: bio-chemical, pharmacological and structure—activity relationships. New York: Alan R Liss; 1986. p. 545-58.

Wahren J, Denis J, Desurmont P, et al. Is intravenous administration of branched chain amino acids effective in the treatment of hepatic encephalopathy? A multicenter study. *Hepatology* 1983; 3: 475-80.

Wang CB, Chang AM. Plasma thromboxane B2 changes in severe icteric hepatitis treated by traditional Chinese medicine—dispelling the pathogenic heat from blood, promoting blood circulation and administrating large doses of radix Paeoniae—a report of 6 cases. *Chung Hsi I Chieh Ho Tsa Chih* 1985; 5: 326–8, 322 [in Chinese].

Wang Y, Ma R. Effect of an extract of *Paeonia lactiflora* on the blood coagulative and fibrinolytic enzymes. *Chung Hsi I Chieh Ho Tsa Chih* 1990; 10: 70, 101–2 [in Chinese].

Watanabe K, Fujino H, Morita T, et al. Solubilization of saponins of Bupleuri radix with ginseng saponins: Cooperative effect of dammarene saponins. *Planta Med* 1988; 54: 405–8.

Wichtl M. *Herbal Drugs and Phytopharmaceuticals*. Boca Raton, FL: CRC Press, 1994, 486–9.

Xue JX, Jiang Y, Yan YQ. Effects of the combination of *Astragalus membranaceus* (Fisch.) Bge. (AM), root of *Angelica sinensis* (Oliv.) Diels. (TAS), *Cyperus rotundus* L. (CR), *Ligusticum chuanxiong* Hort. (LC) and *Paeonia veitchii* Lynch (PV) on the hemorrheological changes in normal rats. *Chung Kuo Chung Yao Tsa Chih* 1993; 18: 621–3, 640 [in Chinese].

Yamamoto M, Kumagai A, Yamamura Y. Structure and actions of saikosaponins isolated from Bupleurum falcatum L. I. Anti-inflammatory action of saikosaponins. *Arzneim Forsch* 1975; 25: 1021–3.

Yamamoto S, Oka H, Kanno T, et al. Controlled prospective trial to evaluate Shosaiko-to in preventing hepatocellular carcinoma in patients with cirrhosis of the liver. *Gan To Kagaku Ryoho (Jpn J Cancer Chemother)* 1989; 16: 1519–24 [in Japanese].

Yamashiki M, Nishimura A, Nomoto M, et al. Herbal medicine sho-saiko-to induces tumor necrosis factor-alpha and granulocyte colony-stimulating factor in vitro in peripheral blood mononuclear cells of patients with hepatocellular carcinoma. *J Gastro Hepatol* 1996; 11: 137–42.

Yamashita JI. Effect of Tsumura skakuyaku-kanzo-to on pain at muscle twitch during and after dialysis in the patients undergoing dialysis. *Pain and Kampo Medicine* 1992; 2: 18–20.

Yang DG. Comparison of pre- and post-treatment hepatohistology with heavy dosage of Paeonia rubra on chronic active hepatitis caused liver fibrosis. *Chung Kuo Chung Hsi I Chieh Ho Tsa Chih* 1994; 14: 195, 207–9 [in Chinese].

Zhang Y. The effects of nifedipine, diltiazem, and *Paeonia lactiflora* Pall. on atherogenesis in rabbits. *Chung Hua Hsin Hsueh Kuan Ping Tsa Chih* 1991; 19: 100–3 [in Chinese].